BOOB IN A BOX

A Guide for Anyone Having a Mammogram

By
A.J. Funstuff

Boob in a Box
Copyright © 2017
A. J. Funstuff
All Rights Reserved.
ISBN: 978-1-980-32452-2
In compliance with Amazon Kindle Direct Publishing Terms of Service and except as permitted under the U.S. Copyright Act of 1976, no part of this work may be reproduced, distributed, or transmitted in any form or by any means, or stored in a database or retrieval system, without prior written permission of the author.
Disclaimer: The information provided in this publication is designed to provide some entertaining and helpful insights on the subjects therein. The contents are not meant to be used, nor should it be used to diagnose or treat any medical condition. For any medical concerns, please consult your own physician. Amazon Kindle KDP and the author are not responsible for any damages or

negative consequences from any treatment, action, application or preparation to any person reading or following the information in this publication. References are provided for informational purposes only and do not constitute endorsement of any websites or other sources. Readers may find a website has changed URLs and should consult a search engine if a site is not found. Ensure the **NCX view** is enabled in the **Go To Menu** of your Kindle device/application.

* * *

Contents

Boob in a box 1
PART 1: THE MAMMO SQUISH 2
PART 2: THE WAITING ROOM 5
PART 3: HOUSTON, WE HAVE A PROBLEM 10
PART 4: INHERITED TRAITS 15
PART 5: YOU WANT A PIECE OF ME? 20
PART 6: I NEED A WHAT? 27
PART 7: I HATE SURPRISES 38
PART 8: WHAT KIND OF BREAST CANCER DID THEY FIND? 45
PART 9: WHAT ELSE DON'T THEY TELL YOU? 48
PART 10: SURVIVING AND LIVING 55
PART 11: Other Sources 58
PART 12: EPILOGUE 62

※ ※ ※

Dedicated to all those who have anxiously waited to learn the outcome of a mammogram.*

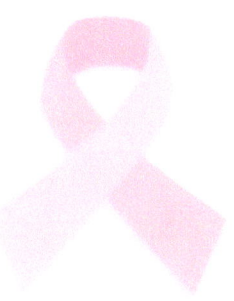

*A mammogram is a standard screening test for breast cancer and is an x-ray of our boobs. They position each one, in turn, between two plates that squish it. The squish reminds me of my waffle iron. Fortunately, they don't use a waffle iron to take a mammogram. Hold your breath. Don't move...OUCH. Breathe.

PART 1: THE MAMMO SQUISH

I have been that lady sitting next to you in the mammogram waiting room. You should know that I am not a trained medical professional but wish to share my treatise on how to treat us. It is about keeping your sense of self-empowerment and, especially, keeping your sense of humor. There are some things you can't keep, like that lovely exam gown they provide as you wait for your mammogram results, but many things are in your power.

  I have been in this waiting room each year for the last nineteen years. The radiologist who reads my mammogram today compares this scan with a prior scan to see if something has changed that would justify getting a closer look. If this is your first time or you've been here before, the best thing to do is keep a positive attitude. Ever notice how the word "tit" is right in the middle of the word "at**tit**ude"? There's something to be said for that. But to stay positive, you must educate yourself and keep driving for the answers that make sense to you if your latest mammogram is flagged.

In the telling of my "Boob in a Box" story, I put in some "what-if-they-find-something" advice. Truly, breast cancer is a serious subject but humor and a keen understanding will help you to get through it. This booklet may answer some questions. Isn't that why you picked it up?

Perhaps this is your regular yearly *screening* mammo. It is good you're here to get checked out. Maybe it is a *diagnostic* mammo for something that is bothering you such as unexplained pain, lumps, unusual nipple discharge, dimpling of the skin or something else. If you see or feel something out of the ordinary, blowing it off as "probably nothing" is not the advice you would give to your best friend. Either way, this is an unsettling day.

    My story is meant to inspire you to advocate for yourself. What I offer here is what happened with me and — be prepared — it isn't pretty. Your journey will be different and unique to you. Still, you may wish to e-mail me if this was helpful or if you simply wish to say you find my humor annoying. Either way, I'd like to know and will be happy to answer you if you provide your name and e-mail.

You may reach me at ajfunstuff@comcast.net.

* * *

PART 2: THE WAITING ROOM

That exam gown ... well, maybe no one told you at the time, but when you have it on, you look gorgeous. There we all are, sitting side-by-side-by-side in these lovely garments. I have been there with other women in the waiting room; some old, some late-fifties, some middle-aged and maybe even a twenty-something. It levels the playing field of class, age, race and religion to a commonality of sisterhood as we wait together. We hope there is nothing to worry about other than the fashion statement we're making.

We eye each other as we bide our time, like horses in the confines of the starting gate at the Kentucky Derby, waiting for our release. We hope they will send us back into the wild with nothing to worry about. Instinctively, we know it can go either way when our name is called.

So there I am, waiting for the mammogram results in that snazzy gown. My mind wanders, thinking how this is like being in the car dealership waiting room. I figure they'll tell me that I passed my annual inspection, the chassis is in pretty good shape for its age, and I am free to go. I just need to remember to come back for an oil change in 3,000 miles. What I didn't want to hear is that the transmission is shot.

I am thinking they must be done by now so I can go home...unless it is bad news. Maybe not. Maybe they are being extra careful. After all, reading a mammogram is not as clear-cut as determining if you need new brake pads.

I am told that even a 3-D Digital Tomosynthesis image can be tricky to interpret if you have dense breast tissue or fibrocystic breast tissue (benign lumps); that was me. I was told this is nothing to worry about — I figure lots of women have dense breast tissue who never get cancer. After going through the annual squish, I never imagined this year's mammogram would be any different.

As I wait, I think back to my youth. I may have been the first girl in school to get a bra and ditch the undershirt. In junior high, the boys teased me and said they could see me coming around the corner before I actually came around the corner. My boobs grew to a size 42DD by the eighth month of my pregnancy. My hubby loved them more than I did. I was tired of pummeling my chest with my knees every time I would get on the exercise bike.

Why is it taking so long to get my results? Maybe I should start to worry now. I'll wait two more minutes. Okay, how about now? Should I start to worry now? Hey, how come she got to leave and I am still here? I was here long before she arrived! Maybe I should start to worry.

With the "thumbs' up," I can escape to where I stowed my clothes and shed the fears along with that darling exam gown and get back to my life. Each year, I would feel a sense of relief as I'd leave the medical facility, happy I dodged that bullet. Geez, what is taking so long?

Early detection is the first line of defense against breast cancer. I need to trust them when they tell me that I am in the clear...or if they are not sure and need to ask me to go through another test, like an ultrasound or even a biopsy. I realize *they want to be sure* they didn't miss anything. It is important to get the "all clear" and if that means another squish, so be it, right? Now is the time to be a cooperative patient and wait and see.

Almost every day, we are reminded to take good care of our health. We are bombarded with messages on radio and TV ads sponsored by pharmaceutical companies, our local healthcare system, or the American Cancer Society. We also have well-meaning family members who do not want to have to pick up the slack for all the stuff we do if we're out of commission. Granted, it is nice to be needed. And while it is nice to hear our families say, "be well" and "take care," I believe we try to stay well because we know they can hardly function without us.

So there we are, alone in our thoughts in that waiting room. Someone who came with us today may be out at the front desk waiting area but right now it's just you, me, and the other ladies in those exam gowns in that back waiting room. As comedian Jerry Seinfeld said, "There's no chance of not waiting...that's the name of the room."1

We will all get through this, but the suspense is killing me. I think I will start to worry now. I wonder if all the other women are worrying, too, as they flip the pages of their long-expired magazines. No one says a word. We all are a little uncomfortable as we wait for our name to be called.

* *

PART 3: HOUSTON, WE HAVE A PROBLEM

They finally call my name and this is the first time I am ushered into a darkened room with computer monitors showing the mammograms from today's patient load. The radiologist wants me to see my own images to show me something. My worry meter is starting to sound an alarm.

    I sit down next to the doctor of radiology and notice the outline of the general shape of a squished boob and a bunch of white dots scattered throughout the image like stars in the night sky. I look at the screen and think I might as well be viewing an image from the Hubble telescope. The radiologist points to a hazy cluster that reminds me of the Andromeda nebula, a spiral galaxy 2.5 million light-years from earth. My ADD (attention deficit disorder) has me distracted as I try to see if that is my name in the corner of the screen. I need reassurance that she has a picture of the right lady.

The radiologist tells me one area seems suspicious and recommends a biopsy, which is where they take a little tissue sample to be viewed under a microscope in a Pathology lab to determine if there are cancer cells in my breast tissue.

I do not feel any lump. Of course, I haven't been good about doing monthly self-breast exams.

The radiologist explains the dots, known as micro calcifications, may be nothing but could turn out to be DCIS (ductal carcinoma *in situ*, Stage 0 breast cancer). Only a pathology report from a properly executed biopsy can tell the story. Stage Zero is the first in a succession of five stages of breast cancer so I know that if it is cancer, they caught it early. I must not neglect this. I have to face the fear, which I have going in for a mammogram in the first place. Since I need a biopsy, I agree to become a human pin-cushion to see what the dots are all about.

I am given a brochure that says most biopsies show no cancer is present but they want me to have it scheduled right away. There's a mixed message if ever there was one! All I could do was take the brochure and go through the motions to do what had to be done. I ditched the exam gown, got dressed, and made the biopsy appointment at the front desk.

Could this be your next mammogram scenario? Will you go in scared or empowered by knowing what to expect next? Please read on just in case today's mammogram finds something unexpected as it did for me.

If you are told you need more views, they may want to do another mammogram, an ultrasound, or go forward with a biopsy as the next step.

Ask if your facility offers a 3-D mammogram, known as Digital Tomosynthesis. (Be sure your insurance will cover it). It's the latest machine for mammography though it can also miss stuff since all machines have their limitations. Sometimes it is the radiologist who misses stuff and not the machine, but when new technology does a better job, isn't it time to move forward and ditch the old? Is anyone still using a mimeograph machine instead of a copier? Did the Smithsonian run out of space for outmoded items?

To be fair, 3-D is not yet in standard use at all mammography screening centers. The older machines can help radiologists get enough information to recommend further testing if they spot something on the film. With one in eight American women getting breast cancer, it is important to know the state of your breast health.

If you are under age forty-five and are not in the waiting room as you are reading this, you probably never had a mammogram but may worry you need one. Insurance companies may not cover a screening mammogram this early in your life but some women in their twenties and thirties have had breast cancer. As one support group's slogan says, "Fight like a girl." If you suspect something is not right and you're running into a road block because of your age, *DEMAND* that your primary care doctor or gynecologist order a mammogram because you found something new. You know your own body best and if something isn't right, you need to speak up and empower yourself by getting the attention you deserve from your primary care physician (PCP) or a gynecologist. Trust me when I tell you that it is easier to deal with cancer than to navigate the system that serves cancer patients.

Yes, they saw something they didn't like on my mammogram and today I am a cancer survivor. I have to admit losing a breast was traumatic but it is not the worst thing in the world. The actual "boob in a box," that silicone breast form to keep me from toppling over to the right, gets stuffed inside a specially pocketed bra during the day and, at night, it rests in a pretty pink, zippered, round case that looks like a hat box. It inspires me to tell you my thesis on my prosthesis. One mystery to me is why the manufacturer felt a woman would want a pretend nipple poking through her clothing.

While you're waiting on your mammogram results, let's talk a little bit about genes.

* * *

PART 4: INHERITED TRAITS

People talk about the nice aspect of genetics when someone says you have your mother's eyes or grandmother's beautiful complexion. These are the traits easily seen which you are glad you inherited. There are other genes you may have inherited but cannot know about which could spell a predisposition for developing breast cancer. Getting genetic testing is a consideration if you know that cancer runs through your family tree. If you carry a genetic risk, it may guide your decisions about your breast healthcare.

    A decade earlier, I participated in a clinical trial and tested negative for two of the breast cancer genes (BRCA1/BRCA2). Great, I thought. I have a lower risk of getting breast cancer because I don't have those genes, though genetics are only part of the equation. Environmental exposure to toxins can have as much to do with it as other factors like obesity, alcohol consumption, x-ray exposure, birth control, something in the water, or the hormones given to livestock that end up in our dinner. Look at http://www.cancer.org to learn more about risk factors.

Even though other women in my family tree had breast cancer, for all I know, my getting it might have had something to do with living too close to Three-Mile Island nuclear plant which had a near melt-down. Maybe I ate too many processed foods. Who knows? If your insurance will cover genetic testing, why not go for it? If you have kids, it could be helpful to know if you passed along undesirable genetic material along with your pretty eye color. Be advised that men can get breast cancer, too.

As to my family history, my mother had a small cancerous tumor in one breast. She did not go through genetic testing because it wasn't available last century. The tumor was found early in the game, and she had a lumpectomy with radiation. I remember her showing me how her otherwise pale skin had turned to a red breast from the treatments; she said she was glad her name wasn't Robin. She had a pretty good sense of humor. She lived many years after that surgery, later dying from an overdose of French fries and ice cream.

On my father's side, his mother died at age forty-four of breast cancer. I never got to meet her and, for some reason, I was named after her. I am not superstitious but I think my father would have served me better to name me after someone who had a long and healthy life...but maybe I am over-thinking this because a genetic component had been ruled out.

The directive from the American Cancer Society (ACS) is to begin getting yearly mammograms from a baseline of age forty-five. ACS revised their guidelines in 2015, saying screening is optional for ages forty to forty-five.

If you are younger than the guidelines and are reading about breast cancer because of a strong family history, you can look into genetic testing. If you test positive for the BRCA gene mutation, check with your insurance provider to see if you can get screened earlier and cover the cost or try to find a free clinic.

Actress Christina Applegate, at age 36, was diagnosed with cancer through an MRI test and had a bilateral (both sides) prophylactic mastectomy. She had the BRCA gene mutation, her mother had breast cancer, and she started screenings at age 30. Younger women have dense breasts so standard mammograms may not be able to detect an early growth. That is why Ms. Applegate got the MRI but that is not the standard of care. She had to push for that. As a result of the roadblocks she experienced, she started a foundation to help pay for this vital diagnostic tool needed by young, high-risk women. To learn more, you can visit:

http://www.rightactionforwomen.org

or www.youngsurvival.org/breast-cancer-in-young-women. These resources recognize younger women have a statistically higher cancer rate than in years past, particularly among African-American women.

I am 59 years old at this point and I am worried about going through a biopsy, not so much for whatever they do to get a biopsy done, but what they will find and all the unknowns ahead of me. The day of my biopsy is on my calendar. I arrange for the day off work and plan on going alone. There is no reason to have anyone with me since it is not going to be anything major. A little pinch and it'll be over.

* * *

PART 5: YOU WANT A PIECE OF ME?

I learned there are different methods of doing a biopsy. However they do it, the radiologist will be able to see the inside of you in real time as they use a gizmo to get a little tissue sample out from (hopefully) just the right spot. Some biopsies are taken while you are lying on your back. They numb the breast and an ultrasound-guided needle biopsy is done to obtain the sample of suspicious breast tissue. In my case, I get to go through a stereotactic biopsy. I do not know the medical justification for this method over the other method and, frankly, I am not interested to know.

    For my procedure, they numb my left breast and then it pops through a hole in a rather uncomfortable exam table as I lay on my stomach.

The underside of the table is a mammogram squish and a special gizmo guided by the radiologist who then takes a small sample of suspected cancerous breast tissue out while leaving behind a clip, which is a *really tiny* titanium metal shape.

Do not be alarmed; the ones shown here are larger than actual size.[2]

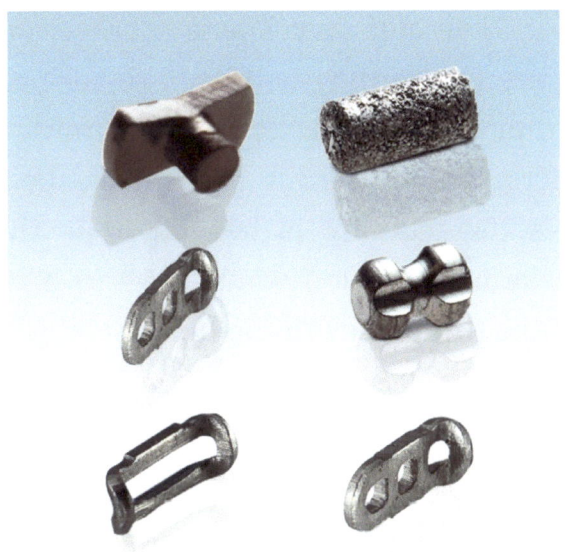

In either case, you only feel a little pressure and no pain until it's all over and the numbness wears off. You can have Tylenol® or other acetaminophen pain reliever. You might bruise at the biopsy site and they give you a miniature ice pack to minimize that. Mine immediately defrosted but they can be frozen again and again. Ask for two of them so you can keep swapping them out from the freezer.

The pathologist (a special doctor who looks at cells under a microscope in a pathology lab) gets the tissue sample and can determine if cancer is there or not.

The clip serves as a marker for the surgeon to see where they will need to surgically remove a tumor if cancer is found, assuming you and the doctor agree to a lumpectomy as being sufficient. If a mastectomy is needed or is the choice you make because you want to remove it entirely, the whole thing goes to the lab.

There is a possibility another lump is in the breast that was not previously detected (or biopsied) that would be found by pathology since they rake through all the tissue they get and they will report the location of the embedded clip and its proximity to any other cancerous tissue they find.

If the biopsy comes back negative for cancer, this marker shows up on future mammogram films and the radiologist will know you had a prior biopsy and will watch this area a little closer.

Each time they take a biopsy sample, the new area gets a different-shaped clip which is why there is a variety of them. If you get more than one biopsy, they have to see what shape was already put in so they select a different one.

Rest assured, you won't feel the clip in you and it should not set off the alarms at the airport. If it did, the TSA agent could not grope you enough to feel the metal clip. You can ask for a card from the doctor or some kind of note if you fear the airport security doesn't believe you.

Lucky you…it is good news and the pathology report says everything appears benign. Fewer women get diagnosed with Stage 0 (zero) than with higher stages because it is very hard to catch it early when a tumor is less than one centimeter. Maybe, like me, you didn't learn the metric system in school. We know inches. How big is a centimeter?

There are 2-1/2 centimeters per inch. The thing is, when it comes to cancer, we have zero tolerance for errors, but it happens. They can miss taking the biopsy from the place where there is cancer, just misjudging it by a tiny bit, and then reporting what turns out to be a "false negative." This is a very scary prospect since it can be a year before your next mammogram, so we always hope that a biopsy is poking in the right place. Is it wrong to wonder if they missed poking in the right place? This is a valid concern because people are human and mistakes can be made. They made mistakes with me but I am told it is highly unusual for that to happen. Lucky me.

As I brace for my biopsy, I notice a radio playing Elton John's, "Don't Go Breaking My Heart." I'm thinking, "Don't go poking my boob." I sang it out loud and the two assistants in the room laughed. I get more silly than usual when I am nervous. I don't think the radiologist laughed. She is a very serious person.

Of course, now I will never be able to hear that Elton John song again and not think about that moment. They should play some obscure elevator music or relaxing instrumental. This is not the time to hear the traffic report or have them ruin one of your favorite songs. If you feel comfortable enough to ask, suggest they turn the radio off before you get started.

A week later, I get notified that I have to go back for a second stereotactic biopsy. The one they took was near the chest wall and now they want another one near the nipple. I go through that again, getting another clip. Now I am on edge, waiting for the second report. A few days pass before I receive a call from the breast imaging center telling me the news. Both biopsies confirmed DCIS Stage 0 throughout my left breast. My initial mental ability to process the fact that I am diagnosed with breast cancer is disorienting. I am told to meet with a surgeon to figure out the next step.

I am angry. If the whole boob is full of cancer, I am thinking I may have to lose that breast altogether. Geez, a mastectomy! ME! Half-crazed, half-joking, I threaten to drive past Hooters[3] restaurant and shoot the "**s**" off their sign. If I am going down one boob, I am going to take them down with me.

I begin acting weird. At the grocery store, I see a man in the produce department holding a cantaloupe in each hand and I said to him, "Nice melons, guy!" I was out of control. Getting a diagnosis of breast cancer put me in an unimaginable funk. I will tell you that after the initial shock, you get past that angry stage and when all is said and done, you can be glad that you went for that mammogram screening to take care of your health and your life. You still there in the mammogram waiting room?

    Remember to ask your physicians all the questions you can think of, every step of the way. And, be advised, some information on the Internet may be questionable so if you do any research, be sure it is from a reliable source. You will find some resources from professionals at the end of this story.

* * *

PART 6: I NEED A WHAT?

Now I have to "shop" for a breast surgeon. I hear good things about one female surgeon at a nearby hospital. In part, I choose her because she is younger and consistency in my care is important. I thought it best to pick someone more likely to outlive me than the other way around. An older, highly recommended surgeon was rumored to retire soon. I did not want to start with one and have to switch down the road. One other doctor also comes highly recommended but is said to have "a cowboy mentality." I don't know what that means. I think a woman's delicate, surgically skilled hands may be better than someone who can lasso a steer. I make the appointment with my first choice.

My family comes to my appointment so everyone will know the game plan. I want more sets of ears to absorb whatever she is going to tell me since I am still reeling from the initial news.

I have heard the word "mastectomy" before. I wish to clarify that one should not mispronounce mastectomy. If you've been saying, "**mass**-ek-toe-me," that is a made-up word that could describe what you call the action of a mother removing her loudmouth kid from the sanctuary during church mass services. Properly pronounced "mass-**tect**-o-me," it is the operation to surgically remove the entire breast and selected lymph nodes when diagnosed with cancer.

This is not to be confused with a "lump-**ek**-toe-me" which is where both a tumor and some surrounding healthy and normal tissue (known as the margins) are removed along with selected lymph nodes, keeping most of you intact.

If the whole breast is removed as a preventive measure, this surgical procedure is pronounced "pro-fill-lack-tik." Prophylactic mastectomy can be a choice if genetic testing indicates you have the BRCA1 and/or BRCA2 gene mutation since this increases the risk that, one day, you may get breast cancer. Movie stars Christina Applegate and Angelina Jolie did that. It gave them peace of mind and it is an option you can talk about with a cancer genetics counselor and a breast surgeon.

If any women in your family (mother, sister, or aunt) have been diagnosed with breast cancer and you carry the gene mutations, it is good to be concerned about your own risk factors for getting breast cancer and consider prophylactic mastectomy, even if your mammograms have been okay. There are always risks and you must weigh all the factors carefully.

So here I am, listening to the surgeon say I have no choice and the whole left boob has to go. I don't think I heard much after that. It doesn't seem real that I need to face a decision about how to get another boob in its place. I am just thankful I am not a pooch with eight of these things!

I decide to call a mastectomy being "dis-com-**boob**-u-lated" (another made-up word). I told you I joke more when I am nervous.

Even though it is horrible news, my breast surgeon gives me a hug and reassures me that she

will help me get through this. She gives me three choices:
- Left breast mastectomy and while I am still on the operating table, the plastic surgeon would double-team the operation immediately following the breast removal to do the reconstruction by inserting an expander to make room for an implant at a later date.
- Left mastectomy with reconstruction later. A plastic surgeon can do this a year down the road or ten years down the road and, by law, it would still be covered by insurance.
- Left mastectomy and no reconstruction. A prosthetic in my bra would even me out so my clothes fit right and so I don't make right turns all day.

I try to focus on what I want to do. I feel pressured to make a choice on the spot. The breast surgeon tells me to think it over but I have thought of little else for the last month since the first pathology report issued.

Do I want an artificial implant? Would I prefer some other kind of plastic surgery where my own body tissues can be relocated to my chest to fill out the bra without anything artificial inside me (options have the word "flap" in them)? What are the pros and cons of each surgical reconstruction operation? How disfiguring might the end result be? Will I need chemo or radiation (or both) and can that delay the reconstruction? How will I cope in the meantime? Since I will need to conceal the disfigurement of a mastectomy, even if only for a few months until I am able to have reconstruction, can I handle that? How can I choose what to do and continue to hold my job? Do I consider going flat with the removal of the right healthy breast at the same time?

I am a control freak and was wading through a ton of information (one needs hip boots). I have to select the path forward. My husband and I decide to get a second opinion about the right breast and if it is okay, maybe it is best to leave it alone, with a tweak of a reduction to even me out. That second opinion did influence me to think that losing one breast was enough.

Do I want a "boob in a box" as a daily reminder for the rest of my life? I'd have to put it away at night in that cute pink hatbox it comes packaged in. Would sleeping be difficult if I only had one breast flopping around? What would I do if I wanted to swim? Would my pretend boob go in the bra of the swimsuit? Would it become a flotation device or pool toy? Could I look at my disfigured lopsided self in the mirror afterwards? So many questions swirled in my head. I have never been in a kayak but, at this moment, it feels like I am in one; there's no paddle and I am heading toward Niagara Falls.

At this initial meeting with the breast surgeon, I did not realize that a bilateral mastectomy was an option. It simply does **_not_** occur to me that I should remove the right breast along with the left one. I decide getting an implant is the way to go, instead of doing the double. I want cleavage and to look as normal as I can — but smaller. Being big-breasted was a strain on my back and it was hard for men to not stare at my ample bosom. I decide reconstruction should make me no larger than a "B" cup.

As I am sitting there, discussing my treatment plan, it occurs to me that I always used to sing "on key" but after the mastectomy, I would be a little flat...at least for a while.

The breast surgeon arranges for me to get an appointment with the plastic surgeon so I could be evaluated and a surgery date set up where they would work in succession in the operating room.

The next day, we meet the plastic surgeon. I let her know I no longer want to be a 42DD and wish to reduce to a "B" cup. She assures me she can make that wish come true. She asks me to be bare-chested and then she takes photos of me from the front and the side, as though I am getting a porno mugshot. Then I put the exam gown back on and we talk. She thinks I am "ahead of the curve" because I have read about all the possible kinds of reconstruction and know I want an implant. The only question I had was whether I wanted saline-filled or a silicone-filled.

Years ago, silicone implants were recalled, just like airbags in cars. They posed a danger if they broke, spilling toxic contents. Today's silicone implants are safe because the substance will not spill if the shell breaks; the gel holds its shape and it may not be discovered until your next check-up. However, if a saline implant shell breaks, you immediately flatten out. That happened to a friend of mine who tripped over her cat and fell. It was truly a deflating experience. Since saline is safe, the liquid is absorbed into body tissues and eliminated naturally. The one thing I did not know is that implants are not guaranteed for life and replacements need to be installed about every ten years.

The plastic surgeon goes on to say I would have to put a prosthetic in a special bra for a few months while I am lopsided. Once the expander reaches the "B" cup size through a series of "fills" and tissues get used to being undisturbed for a while, I would no longer need the "boob in a box". The expander would be replaced by the actual implant at a same-day operation as the breast reduction surgery on my right breast. This can be a six-month process.

She explains how she can fashion nipples from my extra tissues. I read somewhere that there is a small chance that they may not "take" and the tissues may die and fall off (what they call necrosis), so it was my choice not to have them. At age 59, I had no plans to suckle pretend children with pretend nipples. Men use nipples like radio control knobs anyway and since there would be no feeling in the one side, it just seems silly to have them. She would have more leeway in how she would reduce the right breast.

If you opt for nipples, they can look quite natural and you can get a tattoo to get the deeper colored areolas (the darker circle of tissue surrounding the nipples) put on. There are before-and-after pictures the surgeon can show you so you can see how pretend nipples can look. It just wasn't my thing. She was a bit taken aback about my not wanting nipples. I told her my reason: Barbie never needed them and Ken never complained.

The day before my mastectomy, my husband and I met with the plastic surgeon again so she could draw on my body (cut on the dotted line) and go over last minute instructions. She also gave us the prescriptions for pain and the antibiotic to fill the day prior, which was very smart thinking.

Once you start on a certain path with the implant as the end goal, you cannot go back and opt for something else, say a DIEP flap reconstruction. If you tend to be unsure of yourself, this will be a hard process for you. That is why it is critical for you to learn what all the reconstruction options are, grasp the impact of each one, consider your emotions and physical well-being and the decisions will gel and narrow so you can make the choice that will be right for you.

To explain more about the tissue expander, this is a medical device that will make room for a silicone implant; it takes months for the whole process to complete. As soon as the mastectomy is done and I'm still under anesthesia, the plastic surgeon gets to work to insert the expander and then closes up the wound where the boob used to be. The scar will be on the underside of the breast and virtually hidden once all is said and done.

The expander, shown to me in the office, is basically a deflated silicone implant with a little magnetized metal ring surrounding a port. It is there that a syringe with saline may poke through my skin and into the port, allowing the nurse to release the saline into the implant-shaped expander. A magnet placed on top of my skin finds the ring. I make a note to myself that I should probably stay away from refrigerator magnets.

Done right, the "fills" gradually stretch the tissues to form a larger and larger pocket around it as the skin and muscle accommodate it and, at the second surgery, the doctor swaps out the expander for the actual implant.

Upon recovery from this surgery, subsequent "fill" visits at the plastic surgeon's office means 50cc of saline are put in and I found that was enough to deal with. It is okay to tell them you want it to go slower. No question that it can be painful for a day or two after any measure of saline is input.

So with the mastectomy complete and the expander in, I recover at home. Before too long, I get a call from the breast surgeon and she drops a bomb. Pathology found an invasive cancerous tumor located right between the two biopsy clips. That was my first surprise. I don't like surprises.

NOTE: Christina Applegate's website is at the end of this guide along with a great source to explain the various reconstruction methods.

***

PART 7: I HATE SURPRISES

Surprise #1 Radiology poked in the wrong place twice, despite all that imaging and two biopsies. After the mastectomy surgery, pathology reported they found a Stage One .8cm invasive cancer tumor, *mid-point between the two biopsy clips.*

Surprise #2 After finding they missed a tumor in the left breast, I wondered what they missed on the right. Prior to the second surgery where the plastic surgeon would reduce the right breast, I pleaded for a 3-D mammogram and got it done. Then they saw "something" that prompted them to do an ultrasound-guided needle biopsy on the right breast. The "something" is called a hypo-echoic area on the film. The pathology report came up negative. The breast surgeon did not trust that report.

Surprise #3 The day of my final reconstruction surgery, my breast surgeon isn't supposed to be part of this day but she decides that the "something" seen on the right breast 3-D film should be surgically removed ahead of the reduction surgery to be performed by the plastic surgeon. That way they can see what that mysterious "something" is. Another surgeon was pinch-hitting for my regular breast surgeon who was out of town. She cut out some tissue and sent it off to pathology from that area. Pathology found another Stage One tumor in this tissue. So the biopsy was a false negative.

Surprise #4 The surgeon who removed that "something" from my right breast overstepped a line. She announced to my family she didn't think it was anything to worry about. My family was relieved to hear I had no cancer in the other breast. When the pathology report came back, it was verified that another Stage One tumor was found in that right breast tissue. I was able to press an apology out of her to never announce to any family if she thinks she sees or doesn't see cancer. She must wait for the pathology report to come out.

Surprise #5 The day the expander was inserted, 250cc of saline was injected to start. Ouch. It takes many uncomfortable and painful days and nights as the forced expansion of my tissues takes place. My tissues do not like it so they stretch and groan (that was me groaning, too) to accommodate this foreign body. I asked that no more than 50cc at a time of saline be injected per visit. They did not listen to me and put in 60cc one time and 90cc another and it was so uncomfortable because they were stretching it too much at a time. They wanted to speed up the process and I had to suffer for it.

Surprise #6 Now we know the right breast had a malignancy removed, rather inadvertently. I am told that right breast "technically" had a lumpectomy and now I am to be subjected to thirty-three radiation treatments. This would be the "standard of care." I kicked myself for not having a bilateral mastectomy. Now I am on a path that I cannot get off. I cannot refuse the radiation but I tried to quit twice because the pain, redness, and swelling were horrible. Little did I know that was just the beginning of my troubles on my right side.

Surprise #7   The plastic surgeon finished the work but, due to the tumor found in the right breast, the breast surgeon now has to come back and schedule another operation to slit open my armpit to find if a sentinel lymph node "lights up." That means I have to go under general anesthesia again for what is called a lymph node biopsy.

Surprise #8   Once the radiation treatments were over and the swelling went down, a hematoma formed and I had to get 5 successive draining procedures, a sclerotherapy procedure, another surgery to remove the hematoma capsules and lots of damaged tissue (a result of the radiation), the insertion of another drainage tube when a seroma formed, and then a case of radiation recall where the chest skin turned horribly disfigured.

Surprise #9 The right side already had three surgeries, radiation treatment, and many other invasive procedures. The next time a mammogram was due to be had on that remaining breast, an alarmed radiologist wanted me to have an ultrasound and, when that showed something suspicious, I was scheduled for a biopsy again. Back at that same table where I had heard Elton John's song, the radiologist poked in two places, putting in clips in each site.

Surprise #10 I decided on a fourth surgery. I no longer could take any more of this and arranged to have the implant pulled out from the left and a mastectomy of the right breast. I was happy to go totally flat and never need a mammogram again. Emotionally and physically, I was exhausted. I kick myself for not opting for the double mastectomy from the beginning, but I did not have the correct information about the presence of invasive tumors in both breasts. I could only go on the information I had at the time. That is all anyone can do in this difficult decision-making process.

Allow me to repeat that what happened to me was considered highly unusual. Each breast cancer case is totally unique.

Your own path may seem to be a dark and foreboding forest ahead but as you travel through and stake out your guideposts, they will illuminate your path as you go along. Courage is not a trait one has but is what one acquires when you prepare for the unknown.

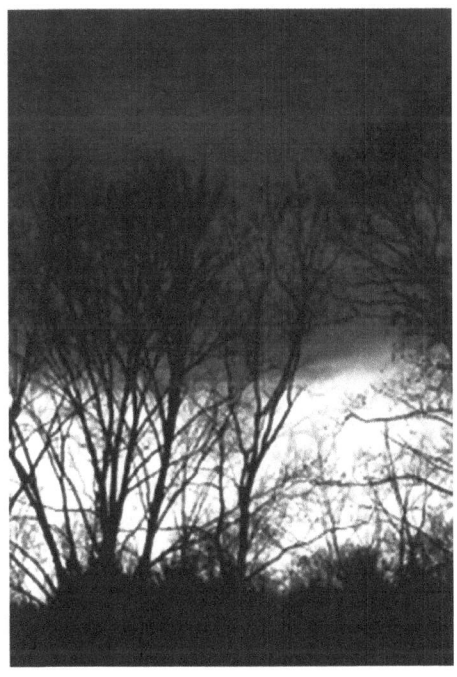

I can only characterize my feelings as having felt betrayed, in part, by the mammography technology itself and mostly by the radiology doctors who read the films and missed the mark when they performed my biopsies. Now you know, even at one of the best hospitals in the USA, it is an imperfect process.

* * *

PART 8: WHAT KIND OF BREAST CANCER DID THEY FIND?

When we see a mutt, some pet owners may say their dog is a "Heinz 57" because it is unknown how many different breeds of pooch make up that dog. From where I sit, it seems that breast cancer is at least as complex to figure out.

Your breast cancer doctor looks at the factors which make up your particular cancer to create the game plan to get your health restored. The treatment may be different for everyone and different medical oncologists may have different ideas about the best way to help you beat the cancer. You can skip this part if you don't want to know what details may make up your particular cancer.

I am aware that decision-making can be hard for some people. I personally have trouble making up my mind about what to make for dinner so getting a handle on what is the best option for cancer care is a bit trickier. Luckily, you have put yourself in the hands of someone who knows what they are doing. Here is a list of some basic information you and your doctor could discuss:

- The current Stage of the cancer (size of the tumor). Stage zero for ductal carcinoma *in situ*; Stage I is 2cm or less; Stage II is 2-5cm; Stage III is larger than 5cm; Stage IV means it has invaded other organs or bones.
- How aggressive the cancer is (based on Ki67 testing). Let's hope it is slow-growing.
- The hormonal nature of the cancer and if it is positive or negative for these (estrogen, progesterone, HER-2/neu). One in ten women are triple negative.
- The location of the tumor

- Are the sentinel lymph nodes unaffected or are involved and if so, how many were removed (sentinel node biopsy or axillary lymph node dissection) to gauge the risk of something called lymphedema.

Everyone is different and the doctor will tell you the treatment scenarios tailor-made for your case. One unfortunate factor has to do with your insurance coverage. Will it pay for everything without bankrupting you? After dealing with the diagnosis, the last thing you want to hear is how much this will cost. It is a good idea to get in touch with the financial people at the institution where your surgery will take place to determine your coverage.

* * *

PART 9: WHAT ELSE DON'T THEY TELL YOU?

These are things no one talks about until way down the road. Maybe you do not want to hear these details but here you are, waiting on those mammogram results, year in and year out and it is good to know what you could possibly have to face.

- Lymph nodes and the risk of lymphedema

Surgeons biopsy the sentinel lymph nodes and remove a number of them during the surgery and if they are clear, you can count yourself very lucky. If they have to take out many of them to help reduce the chances of recurrence and metastatic cancer, you face a lifetime of being careful that no blood pressure cuff or injection takes place on that arm to help avoid the chance of getting lymphedema. You need to avoid getting sunburned, cut, burned, or otherwise injured. Some say even air travel can bring it on. If you get lymphedema, you may need to stop wearing rings, watches, and bracelets and start wearing a compression sleeve. One great site to learn more about this is http://www.lymphedivas.com/

- Nerve damage and numbness that may never go away

You may have nerves cut and lose feeling so that shaving under your arm must be done with an electric shaver rather than a disposable blade because you can cut your skin and not even know you're bleeding.

- Hormone side effects

You need to determine the worth of the percentage points between survival with or without the pills. The medical oncologists will give you some "odds." Tamoxifen is generally given to pre-menopausal women while generic Anastrozole (for the prescription equivalent Arimidex®) is more often given to post-menopausal women. I determined I would not take the medicine that they wanted me on for five to ten years. They talk about survival rates for five years out since that is where the statistics can best be interpreted.

One of the side effects listed on the Anastrozole hand-out said "vision problems." That really caught my attention. This medicine can cause traction of the eye and since I already have posterior vitreous detachment and lattice degeneration of the retina, I flagged this side effect to my ophthalmologist and in doing research on Pub-Med, determined it was risky for me to start the hormone therapy. I said I would rather fight cancer twice than become a blind woman.

- Radiation treatments

You can get 100% Aloe Vera gel from a company called Fruit of the Earth. I found it is available at several retailers. It is a natural substance to soothe burned skin. Since you will need follow-up care, think about if you have to go many miles away to get to those appointments.

Radiation is a daily trip for 33 sessions (except for weekends). If you're living in an area where winter weather, transportation issues, or other factors could get in the way of your treatment plan, then you may need to consider all those logistics.

- Chemotherapy treatments

Chemo rounds (how many sessions and timing in-between each session) vary so this will be different for different people. One thing I did not have was chemo so I am less familiar with it. There are pills and some treatments are given through an intravenous (IV) line. Since veins can have a hard time taking in the chemo, a port may be installed in your chest to make administering the chemotherapy easier on you. Some therapies may give you mouth sores or a host of other side effects. With some chemo, foods may taste metallic so use plastic utensils to lessen that affect.

- Exercise

Your range of motion will be affected by the surgery and adhesions (scar tissue) may form inside your body that can restrict movement later. Ask for physical therapy and massage therapy for getting your body back to functioning as it did before the surgery. Initially, after surgery, you are warned not to lift more than five pounds. If shopping alone at the grocery store, you can ask the check-out lady to weigh every loaded bag on the produce scale before putting the bags in your cart so you don't hurt yourself loading the bags into your car.

- Wigs and prosthetics

There may be a store near you or shop online where you can find hats, head scarves, wigs, wig liners, wig shampoo for the acrylic fiber wigs, and wig stands to put them on while you sleep. Human hair wigs cost more and require the same attention as real hair but the acrylic ones I found to be natural looking, always hold their style, and are easier to care for. You can get a prescription for the prosthetics from your doctor that will defray or totally cover the costs, depending on your plan. The fake boobs (some call them foobs) pop into the special bras that have pockets to help you fill out your clothes. You can always go flat and not have reconstruction as an option when you make it clear to your breast surgeon that you don't want prosthetics. It can be very liberating to be flat as we were when we were 8 or 9 years old and ran around topless.

- Pink Ribbon

If you didn't already know, the pink ribbon is for the support of those with breast cancer. There are many items available from organizations and retailers that sport the pink ribbon on everything imaginable, particularly in October, which is designated as Breast Cancer Awareness Month. You may find the pink ribbon annoying as it is in your face all month long. Some support groups will give a portion of the profits to support cancer research. Your feelings about announcing to the world that you are a cancer survivor are very personal and maybe you would rather not tell others your story. This is where a support group can help you talk through it. I can tell you from personal experience how nice it is to have a safe place to express the whole range of emotions since everyone there, except perhaps the moderator, is going through it or is a survivor. There are also online support groups, like "What Next" or the private Facebook group "Flat & Fabulous" listed at the end of this guide.

* * *

PART 10: SURVIVING AND LIVING

I do not give myself time to wallow in the "why me" speech anymore because there is no rhyme or reason one person gets cancer and another does not. There will come a time when you will be a few years out from the diagnosis and may not think of yourself so much as a survivor. You will be back to your life. Your perspective will have changed but you are still you.

At the end of the day, it is your body and you need to learn what path makes you feel the most comfortable while reaching for the best survival rate. If you feel like you are being railroaded, ask if this is your only option. If you get an answer that this is the only way that surgeon would go, get a second opinion. You have to totally trust your own instincts and have confidence in the doctors. A different doctor may have a different opinion or have a clinical trial that can be right for you.

So how does one keep a positive attitude? For some it is a deep and abiding faith. For others, it is the support of friends, family and co-workers and cancer survivor support groups. For others, it is the reliance on your own ability to work the system. Sometimes it is a combination of any and all of these. You will need that support because it can be weeks from the time you get the "You've got cancer" call to the time that you have found the right medical team to get you through this and make all the decisions and appointments. You can stew, get angry, or just get busy to learn everything you can to empower yourself. Put your education on the fast-track to eliminate second-guessing yourself and ending up with regrets.

I don't know what tomorrow will bring since I can't find my crystal ball anywhere. I did decide never to wear a bra again and buy lots of pretty lace camisoles and remain flat. That is what I ended up doing and, after all was said and done, I am glad I got that off my chest!

I hope in some small way, my story helps you prepare for what may come your way. If you haven't made the appointment for your annual mammogram, what are you waiting for?

* * *

PART 11: OTHER SOURCES

http://www.langeproductions.com/patient-ed/

Website for the book, "Be a Survivor".[4] I highly recommend you see this book prior to making a decision about your surgery, reconstruction options, and treatment options.

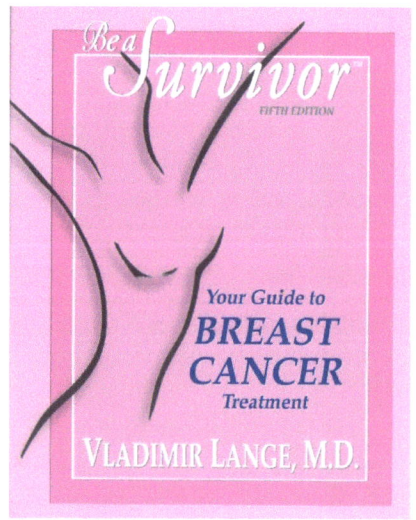

http://www.lookgoodfeelbetter.org An American Cancer Society support organization that can offer you free cosmetics, plus information about wigs and scarves and demonstrated techniques for wearing them in different ways.

http://www.cancer.org
American Cancer Society main website. Also, toll-free 800-227-2345

http://www.whatnext.com An online community of supportive cancer patients where you can pose questions and get advice from others going through it.

http://www.rightactionforwomen.org Founded by Christina Applegate.

https://www.youngsurvival.org/learn Issues around women as young as 18 being diagnosed with breast cancer.

https://www.pubmed.com An online site of abstracts from peer-reviewed medical journals to read about research, chemotherapy trials, information about radiation, and other clinical trial abstracts. The medical journal is sited and you can ask the library for the details

https://ww5.komen.org/BreastCancer/BreastReconstruction.html Susan G. Komen website. Sponsor of "Race for the Cure" and supporter of cancer research programs.

https://soh.hooters.com/Home/ Hooters breast cancer support page. *Hooters also supports breast cancer research in the name of former calendar girl, the late Kelly Jo Dowd, who passed away from breast cancer. One dollar from every Hooters calendar sold goes to research. See their website for details.*

http://www.flatandfabulous.org/ Research your options on reconstruction but know that you do not have to have boobs to feel like a whole woman. This group answers lots of questions if you are considering saving yourself from further surgeries and have it once and done and go flat.

1 Taken from the Jerry Seinfeld comedy CD entitled, "I'm Telling You For The Last Time" track 8. Also on the DVD by the same name.

2 Permission to use the photograph of six biopsy markers courtesy of Hologic LLC.

3 Permission for the use of the Hooters name has been granted by Hooters of America, LLC.

4 Permission to use the front cover graphic of "Be a Survivor" has been granted by Vladimir Lange, MD of Lange Productions.

* * *

PART 12: EPILOGUE

You may be curious how things ended up for me. We're all human...but I expected compassion from the medical community. Unfortunately, that is not always the case. Was there a lawsuit? No. The two-year statute of limitations has now passed and writing this story is helping me to get over the whole thing but I want you to know I am cancer-free.

For me, it is about respect and dignity. The medical community that served me lost sight of what is important and legal action cannot restore that. So far, I have overcome multiple surgeries and treatments but there is one thing I cannot get over — I was banned from the breast imaging center's practice. This was an outrage.

Certainly the radiologist felt bad (and probably embarrassed) that two stereotactic biopsies conducted missed the mark in the left breast and the ultrasound-guided needle biopsy totally missed the cancer diagnosis in the right breast. Mistakes happen and the radiologist must live with those mistakes. In the middle of all this, I heard of a breast cancer seminar held at a local hotel. I attended the conference and sat in the back of the room to learn what doctors say about the state of breast cancer treatment. I got to listen to that radiologist and other doctors I encountered on my journey; breast surgeon, plastic surgeon, radiation oncologist, and medical oncologist. The radiologist called me the next day to tell me our doctor/patient relationship of trust was compromised and I am banned from the imaging practice. I was spotted at the conference according to the health system attorney. The ban is worse than the cancer. I appealed the decision several times but the attorney said it is a lifetime ban and all appeals will be denied. Luckily, I have other places I can go for any future imaging I may need.

✳ ✳ ✳

www.ingramcontent.com/pod-product-compliance
Lightning Source LLC
Chambersburg PA
CBHW040323220526
45473CB00009B/2546